The Power of Genes

Understanding Cancer Risk Through Genetics

by

Sandra R. Trimble

TABLE OF CONTENT

Before deciding to get genetic testing to determine your risk of cancer, it is essential to take into consideration the following factors:

Having an understanding of the test results and the following steps

CHAPTER 6

The prevention of cancer and the treatment of cancer risk

Steps that can be taken to reduce the risk of cancer based on genetic information

How to reduce the risk of cancer through adjustments in one's lifestyle as well as through medical treatment

A complete list of the various screening and preventative measures available for cancer

CHAPTER 7

Conclusion

A synopsis of the most important lessons learned from the book

Definition of some terminologies used in this book

CHAPTER 1

Introduction

The Power of Genes: Understanding Cancer Risk Through Genetics offers a summary of the significance of genetics in determining the likelihood of developing cancer. The readers of this book will gain a better understanding of how genetics can either increase or decrease an individual's risk of developing cancer as a result of the information presented in this text. They will gain an understanding of how to use genetic information to make informed decisions regarding the prevention and management of cancer through the course of a comprehensive discussion of cancer risk, genetic mutations, family history, and testing. Through a better understanding of the role that genetics play, readers of this book will be better equipped to take charge of their own health.

This book is an essential resource for anyone who is interested in gaining a better understanding of how genetics can influence the likelihood that they will develop cancer. They will be able to make a better decisions about their cancer risk and the best way to manage it after gaining knowledge about genetic mutations, family histories, and the various testing options available.

Understanding Cancer Risk Through an Examination of Genetics Through Genetics will provide readers with the knowledge and tools necessary to take an active role in lowering their risk of cancer and living the healthiest life possible.

Understanding Cancer Risk Through an Examination of Genetics, Anyone looking for a helpful resource that provides a comprehensive overview of cancer risk and genetics should look no further than Through Genetics.

At the conclusion of this book, readers will have gained a deeper comprehension of the factors that may increase their likelihood of developing cancer and will be equipped to make well-informed decisions regarding their own health.

A brief overview

The field of study known as cancer genetics examines the hereditary factors that play a role in the development of cancer. It involves looking for mutations in a person's genetic material, both those that are inherited and those that are acquired, that can increase the risk of cancer in that person. Cancer genetics is the study of the relationship between a person's genes and their likelihood of developing cancer, with the ultimate goal of using this information to enhance cancer diagnosis, treatment, and prevention.

This can include investigating genetic mutations that have been linked to particular types of cancer, identifying individuals who are at increased risk due to the genetic background they were born into, and developing new approaches to cancer prevention or management that are based on genetic data.

Explanation of the purpose of the book

This book "The Power of Genes: Understanding Cancer Risk Through Genetics" was written with the intention of enlightening readers regarding the significance of genetics in relation to the risk of developing cancer. The purpose of the book is to provide a comprehensive overview of the subject matter, which will include an explanation of cancer risk, an overview of genetic mutations and their influence on cancer, the significance of being aware of one's family history, and the various options for genetic testing that are currently available.

In addition to this, it provides individuals with actionable advice on how they can utilize their genetic information to reduce their risk of cancer through changes in lifestyle as well as through medical intervention.

The overarching purpose of this book is to equip readers with the knowledge necessary to take charge of their own health by improving their comprehension of the part that genetics plays in determining the likelihood of developing cancer and demonstrating how to use this knowledge to make decisions that are in line with their best interests.

CHAPTER 2

Understanding Cancer Risk

This topic "Understanding Cancer Risk" gives an in-depth explanation of both the concept of cancer risk and the methodology that goes into calculating it. It defines cancer risk as the probability that an individual will be diagnosed with cancer over a predetermined amount of time. This section explains that factors such as lifestyle, exposure to environmental toxins, and genetics all play a role in determining a person's likelihood of developing cancer.

This section of the book also delves into the role that genetics plays in the risk of cancer and explains how genetic mutations can make a person more likely to develop cancer.

Also discusses this chapter is the distinction between inherited mutations and acquired mutations, as well as how the presence of either type of mutation can influence the likelihood of developing cancer. The readers of this book will, by the time they reach the conclusion of this piece, have a crystal clear understanding of what cancer risk is, the factors that contribute to it, and the role that genetics plays in determining an individual's cancer risk.

Definition of cancer risk

A person's likelihood of developing cancer over a given amount of time is referred to as their cancer risk. Cancer risk can also be expressed as a probability. A person's age, lifestyle choices, level of physical activity, medical history of their family, and the presence of genetic mutations all contribute to the likelihood that they will be diagnosed with cancer at some point in their lives. It is possible to estimate the risk of cancer by taking into account all of these factors, which can assist individuals in making wise decisions regarding their health and determining whether or not to take preventative measures to lower their risk of developing cancer. Cancer risk is not a guarantee or a prediction of future health; however, it does provide important information that can be used to guide efforts to prevent cancer and detect it early.

Factors contributing to the development of cancer Risk

A person's likelihood of developing cancer is influenced by a number of different factors, including the following:

1. One's age: As one gets older, their risk of developing cancer goes up.

2. Lifestyle: Factors such as smoking, drinking alcohol, diet, and physical activity can all have an effect on the likelihood of developing cancer.

3. Environmental exposures: Being exposed to particular chemicals, pollutants, or radiation can raise one's risk of developing cancer.

4. A history of cancer in the patient's family: A history of cancer in the patient's family, particularly among first-degree relatives, can indicate an increased risk for certain cancers.

5. Mutations in an individual's genes An individual's risk for developing certain types of cancer may be increased by inherited or acquired mutations in their genes.

It is essential to keep in mind that the risk of developing cancer is not determined by a solitary factor but rather by the interaction of a number of different factors. By gaining an understanding of the factors that raise an individual's risk of developing cancer, one can better direct efforts aimed at cancer prevention and early detection.

How genetics plays a role in cancer risk

The individual's genetic makeup is a major factor in determining their likelihood of developing cancer.

It is possible for a person's risk of developing cancer to be raised by inherited genetic mutations, such as those that can be found in certain syndromes associated with hereditary cancer. Acquired genetic mutations, which can happen throughout a person's lifetime and can be caused by factors such as getting older, being exposed to certain chemicals, or radiation, can also make a person more likely to develop cancer.

Individuals who carry a particular genetic mutation that is known to be linked to a particular form of cancer have an increased likelihood of developing that form of cancer, as does anyone else carrying that mutation.

An increased likelihood of developing breast or ovarian cancer, for instance, has been linked to mutations in the BRCA1 and BRCA2 genes.

When it comes to making informed decisions about one's health and taking actions to reduce the likelihood of developing cancer, it can be helpful to have a thorough understanding of one's genetic history as well as the role that genetics plays in determining the likelihood of developing the disease. This may include increasing cancer screenings, making changes to one's lifestyle, and engaging in preventative interventions such as prophylactic surgery. To lessen the effects of cancer, one of the most important first steps is to gain a better understanding of the role that genetics plays in developing the disease.

What exactly are the genes BRCA1 and BRCA2?

Human genes known as BRCA1 and BRCA2 provide instructions for the production of proteins that play a role in inhibiting the growth of cancerous cells.

The presence of these mutations in an individual's genes can raise that person's risk for developing certain types of cancer, most notably breast and ovarian cancer.

When compared to the average lifetime risk of about 12% for breast cancer and 1.3% for ovarian cancer in the general population, women who have a BRCA1 or BRCA2 mutation have an estimated 55-85% chance of developing breast cancer and a 39% chance of developing ovarian cancer over the course of their lifetime. This is a significant increase from the average lifetime risk of about 1% for ovarian cancer.

The presence of a mutation in the BRCA1 or BRCA2 gene is associated with an increased risk of several other types of cancer, including prostate and pancreatic cancer in males and cancer of the fallopian tube and peritoneum in females.

Individuals who have a history of these cancers running in their families should consider getting tested for BRCA1 and BRCA2 mutations. This testing can provide information about an individual's cancer risk as well as guide efforts to prevent cancer and detect it early.

CHAPTER 3

Cancer Genetics 101
(Fundamentals)

This book "The Power of Genes: Understanding Cancer Risk Through Genetics" contains a section or chapter titled "Cancer Genetics 101," which serves as an introduction to the subject of cancer genetics, at a fundamental level. This section goes over the fundamentals of cancer genetics, such as what cancer genetics is, how genetic mutations can influence the risk of cancer, and the role that genetic testing can play in determining cancer risk and guiding preventative measures.

It is likely that the purpose of the chapter "Cancer Genetics 101" would be to lay a foundation for readers who are new to the subject of cancer genetics by providing them with the fundamental information that is required for them to understand the more complex topics that are discussed later in the book. This section is written in a way that was straightforward and easy to understand, making it an invaluable resource for anyone interested in learning about the connection between genetics and the risk of developing cancer.

An outline of the role that genetic mutations play in the development of cancer

Mutations in an individual's DNA are changes or alterations to the genetic code that can have an effect on that person's health. Some genetic mutations can increase the risk of developing cancer by changing the normal functions of genes that normally work to suppress the growth of cancerous cells. This can lead to an increased likelihood of developing cancer.

Explanation of inherited mutations as well as acquired ones

Inherited mutations and acquired mutations are the two primary categories of genetic changes that can take place.

Inherited mutations are changes or alterations to a person's DNA that are passed down from their parents. These mutations can increase the risk of developing certain types of cancer throughout a person's lifetime. Inherited mutations can be passed down from generation to generation. These mutations are already present in an individual's cells when they are conceived, and they have the potential to be passed on to the individual's offspring.

Acquired mutations, on the other hand, take place over the course of a person's lifetime and are not something that can be inherited from their parents.

Rather, these mutations are as a result of factors such as aging, exposure to particular chemicals or radiation, or errors that take place during the process of DNA replication.

Acquired mutations can build up over time, which can raise the risk of developing cancer by altering the normal functions of genes that normally work to suppress the growth of cancerous cells. Acquired mutations can also increase the likelihood that a person will have cancer. It is essential to keep in mind that an individual's risk of developing cancer can be affected by both inherited mutations and acquired mutations, but the presence of either type of mutation does not necessarily indicate that a person will go on to develop cancer. On the other hand, individuals who are aware of the presence of inherited or acquired mutations may be better equipped to make better choices regarding their health and to take measures that lower their risk of developing cancer.

An increased likelihood of developing breast or ovarian cancer, for instance, has been linked to mutations in the BRCA1 and BRCA2 genes.

When it comes to cancer genetics, genetic testing can be a significant factor in determining an individual's likelihood of developing the disease. Individuals will be able to take measures to lower their risk of developing cancer and undergo increased cancer screenings if they undergo testing to determine the presence of genetic mutations that are associated with an increased risk of developing cancer.

Understanding the part that genetic mutations play in a person's risk of developing cancer is an essential step in mitigating the effects of the disease and enhancing the chances of survival for those who are diagnosed with it.

Different kinds of inherited changes that can make a person more likely to develop cancer.

A person's likelihood of developing cancer can be raised by a variety of genetic mutations, some of which are more common than others. The following are examples of some of the most common mutations that are known to increase the risk of cancer:

1. Mutations in the BRCA1 and BRCA2 genes: There is a correlation between mutations in the BRCA1 and BRCA2 genes and an increased risk of breast and ovarian cancer.

2. Lynch syndrome: Lynch syndrome, also known as hereditary non-polyposis colon cancer (HNPCC), is a genetic condition that raises the risk of developing several different types of cancer, including colorectal, endometrial, gastric, and pancreatic cancers.

3. Li-Fraumeni syndrome: The Li-Fraumeni syndrome is a rare genetic condition that raises a person's risk of developing multiple types of cancer, including sarcomas, leukemia, brain tumors, breast cancer, and adrenocortical carcinoma, among others.

4. Retinoblastoma: Retinoblastoma is a rare form of eye cancer that can be caused by inherited mutations in the RB1 gene.

Retinoblastoma affects only a small percentage of people.

5. Familial adenomatous polyposis (FAP): Familial adenomatous polyposis, also known as FAP, is a genetic condition that raises the likelihood of developing colon cancer.

6. von Hippel-Lindau disease: von Hippel-Lindau disease is a genetic condition that raises the likelihood of developing tumors in various parts of the body, including the eye, the brain, and the spinal cord, among other locations.

It is essential to keep in mind that not all genetic mutations are associated with an increased probability of developing cancer.

While some genetic mutations are harmless and have no effect on an individual's health, others may have a very slight influence on the likelihood of an individual developing cancer.

The presence of a particular genetic mutation does not in and of itself guarantee that a person will develop cancer; however, it can provide important information about the person's cancer risk, which can guide efforts to prevent cancer and detect it at an earlier stage.

CHAPTER 4

Having a good understanding of your family's history

It is possible that an individual's cancer risk can be significantly impacted by the presence of a cancer history in their family. A pattern of cancer developing in multiple members of the same family, frequently spanning multiple generations, is referred to as having a "family history of cancer."

A person's having a history of cancer in their family does not ensure that they will also get cancer, but it does indicate that they may have a higher risk of getting the disease. Because certain cancers have a significant hereditary component and can be passed down from one generation to the next,
it is essential for an individual to be aware of any cancer cases that have occurred within their family.

It is helpful to gather information about the cancer diagnoses and age at diagnosis of your immediate family members (parents, siblings, and children), as well as the diagnoses of any other close relatives, in order to gain a better understanding of the cancer history in your family. Using this information, one may be able to recognize patterns of cancer that might point to an increased genetic risk.

If there is a history of cancer in the individual's family, it may be beneficial to consult with a genetic counselor or a medical professional to discuss the potential implications for the individual's own health as well as the appropriate actions they can take to lower their risk of developing cancer. This may include undergoing genetic testing,
increasing the frequency of cancer screenings, or making adjustments to one's lifestyle. Understanding the history of cancer in your family is an essential step in lowering your own cancer risk and improving your overall health outcomes.

The significance of understanding your family's cancer history

It is important to learn about any history of cancer in one's family for a number of reasons:

1. An increased risk of cancer A family history of cancer can indicate an increased genetic risk for certain types of cancer, which enables individuals to take preventative measures to reduce their risk of developing cancer, such as increasing the number of times they get screened for cancer, making changes to their lifestyle, and getting genetic testing.

2. Early detection Realizing that one's family has a history of cancer can assist an individual in recognizing possible warning signs and in seeking early detection, both of which can improve the individual's chances of successfully undergoing treatment.

3. Personalized treatment plans: If an individual has a family history of cancer, the medical team caring for that individual may take this information into consideration when developing a personalized treatment plan. This is because certain treatments may be more effective based on the individual's genetic background.

4. Empowerment: Knowing the history of cancer in one's family can provide individuals with important information about their health and enable them to take control of their health by allowing them to make informed decisions about the care they receive.

5. Better health outcomes: Early detection and an understanding of an individual's family history of cancer can lead to better health outcomes for that individual. This is because treatment can be initiated earlier, and individuals can take steps to reduce their risk of developing the disease.

A person's overall health outcomes can be improved, and their risk of developing cancer can be reduced, if they are aware of any cases of cancer that have occurred in their family.

How the history of one's family can influence one's likelihood of developing cancer

There are multiple ways in which one's family history can affect their risk of developing cancer:

1. Inherited genetic mutations Certain types of cancer can be caused by genetic mutations that are inherited from one generation to the next. These mutations can be passed down from parent to child. Cancer running in one's family can be an indicator of an increased risk for certain forms of the disease, including breast cancer, ovarian cancer, and colon cancer, amongst others.
2. Environmental and lifestyle factors that are shared by members of the same family Members of the same family frequently share environmental and lifestyle factors that can influence their risk of developing cancer.

For instance, the risk of developing cancer can be increased by smoking, being exposed to environmental toxins, and engaging in unhealthy dietary practices.

3. Increased awareness Having a history of cancer in one's family can increase one's awareness of the disease and encourage them to take preventative measures to lower their risk of developing cancer. These preventative measures can include seeking early detection, making changes to one's lifestyle, and consulting with a genetic counselor or other medical professional.

Early detection: Knowing if there is a history of cancer in one's family can assist an individual in recognizing potential warning signs and seeking early detection, both of which can improve the individual's chances of successfully undergoing treatment.

When it comes to overall cancer risk, an individual's family history of cancer can have a significant impact, and it is essential to take this information into consideration when making decisions about one's own health.

Methods of compiling and interpreting information regarding family history

The following are the steps involved in collecting and analyzing information regarding family history:

1. Collect the necessary information: To begin, it is best to gather information about cancer diagnoses and age at diagnosis by talking to members of the patient's family. This should include the patient's parents, siblings, and children. You can also gather information about any other close relatives, such as grandparents, aunts and uncles, cousins, and other close relatives.

2. Classify the information as follows: Record all of the information that you have gathered, including the type of cancer, the age at which it was diagnosed, and your relationship to the person who has cancer.

In order to better visualize the information, you might find it useful to construct a family tree or make use of a tool such as software designed specifically for family history.
3. Look for patterns: Conduct an analysis on the information that you have gathered to search for patterns of cancer that might point to an increased genetic risk.

For instance, if several close relatives have been diagnosed with breast cancer, this may be an indication of an increased risk for this particular form of cancer.
4. Take into account any other potential risk factors: Take into account any additional risk factors that may have an effect on your likelihood of developing cancer,

such as your age at the time of your first pregnancy, the amount of alcohol you consume, and the amount of exposure you have to toxins in the environment.

5. Consult with a genetic counselor or a medical professional: If there is a history of cancer in your family, it may be beneficial to consult with a genetic counselor or a medical professional in order to determine the potential implications for your health and the appropriate steps you can take in order to lower your risk of developing cancer.

Gathering information about your family's medical history and conducting an analysis of that data is an essential step in lowering one's risk of developing cancer and improving one's overall health. It is essential to acquire as much information as one can and, if necessary, to seek the guidance of a qualified medical expert.

CHAPTER 5

Cancer Risk Evaluation Based on Genetic Testing

An individual's DNA is analyzed during the process of genetic testing for cancer risk in order to determine whether or not they carry any genetic mutations that put them at an increased risk for developing specific types of cancer. This testing can help guide decisions about cancer prevention and early detection, as well as provide important information about an individual's risk of developing cancer.

An overview of the various genetic tests that can be used to assess the risk of cancer

There are a few different genetic tests for determining the likelihood of developing cancer, including the following:

1. Predictive genetic testing: Predictive genetic testing is used to determine if an

individual has a genetic mutation that increases their risk for a particular type of cancer. One example of this would be the BRCA1 and BRCA2 mutations, which are associated with breast and ovarian cancer respectively.

2. Carrier testing: Carrier testing is a type of testing that is used to determine whether or not an individual carries a genetic mutation that could be passed on to their children but does not necessarily increase the individual's own risk for developing cancer.

3. Newborn screening: Newborn screening is a method for identifying certain genetic mutations in newborns that have the potential to cause conditions that are life-threatening.

4. Tumor testing: The purpose of tumor testing is to determine which treatment options are the most effective by analyzing the genetic mutations present in a person's cancer cells.

5. Panel testing: Panel testing is a type of genetic testing that assesses an individual's

risk for several different types of cancer by simultaneously analyzing multiple genes from the individual.

6. Multi-gene panel testing is a type of panel testing that evaluates a large number of genes, frequently dozens or even hundreds, in order to determine an individual's potential risk for multiple forms of cancer.

7. Whole exome or genome sequencing: This type of genetic testing examines an individual's entire exome (the part of the DNA that codes for proteins) or genome (the complete set of DNA in an organism) in order to determine the individual's likelihood of developing multiple forms of cancer and other diseases.

It is essential to have a conversation with a genetic counselor or a qualified medical professional in order to ascertain the kind of genetic testing that would be most suitable for an individual's specific circumstances and to gain an understanding of the potential benefits and restrictions associated with genetic testing.

What to consider before undergoing genetic testing

Before deciding to get genetic testing to determine your risk of cancer, it is essential to take into consideration the following factors:

1. The purpose of the test Although genetic testing can provide useful information about an individual's risk for developing cancer, it is essential to have a clear understanding of both the purpose of the test and the purpose for which the results will be used in order to make informed decisions.

2. The potential drawbacks of testing There are some potential drawbacks to genetic testing, and the results may not provide a comprehensive picture of an individual's risk for cancer.

It is essential to have a solid understanding of the constraints that are imposed by testing as well as what the results can and cannot tell you.

3. The potential for an emotional impact The outcomes of genetic testing may have significant emotional and psychological repercussions; therefore, it is essential to have support and resources at your disposal in order to deal with these outcomes.

4. Maintaining confidentiality is essential, given the potentially sensitive nature of the information gleaned from genetic testing. It is essential to have a clear understanding of how the results will be protected and who will have access to them.

5. Implications for one's health insurance Because genetic testing can be quite pricey, it is essential to have a thorough understanding of how the results may influence one's health insurance coverage and access to medical care.

6. Recommendations for medical care Although genetic testing can help inform medical recommendations for the early

detection and prevention of cancer, it is essential to have a clear understanding of how the results will be applied when making decisions regarding medical care.

7. The availability of resources It is essential to have an understanding of the resources and support that are available, such as genetic counseling, to assist in interpreting the results of genetic testing and in making decisions that are based on accurate information.

Prior to undergoing genetic testing, it is strongly suggested to consult with a genetic counselor or a qualified medical professional.

This will allow individuals to gain a better understanding of the potential benefits and limitations of testing, as well as assistance in weighing the risks and benefits of testing in the context of their own specific circumstances.

Having an understanding of the test results and the following steps

After undergoing genetic testing to determine one's susceptibility to developing cancer, it is critical to not only comprehend the outcomes and what they indicate about one's likelihood of developing the disease, but also the subsequent actions that may be required. The following are some important considerations to keep in mind:

1. The interpretation of the results It is important to have access to a genetic counselor or other medical professional who can help interpret the results of genetic testing and explain what they mean in the context of an individual's specific situation. This is because the results of genetic testing can be difficult to understand, and it is important to have their assistance.

2. A positive test result: If the genetic test reveals a mutation that increases the risk for cancer,
it is important to understand the implications of the results as well as the options for cancer prevention, early detection, and treatment. If the test is positive, it is also important to understand the implications of the results.

3. A negative result from the test: If the genetic test does not uncover a mutation that significantly raises the individual's risk of developing cancer, it is critical to have a thorough understanding of the limitations of the test as well as the implications of the findings for the individual's potential future risk of developing the disease.

4. Confirmatory testing: If the results of a genetic test are unclear or inconclusive, it may be necessary to undergo additional testing in order to confirm the results of the genetic test. In some cases,

it may be necessary to undergo additional testing in order to confirm the results of the genetic test.

5. Recommendations made by medical professionals based on the results of genetic testing Medical professionals may, based on the results of genetic testing, make recommendations for cancer prevention, early detection, and treatment. These recommendations may include making changes to one's lifestyle, undergoing surveillance, or undergoing risk-reducing surgery.

6. Members of the family In the event that the findings of genetic testing reveal a mutation that results in an increased risk of developing cancer, it is essential to consider the repercussions for members of the patient's family and determine whether or not they too may be at an increased risk and require genetic testing.

It is important to work with a genetic counselor or another medical professional in order to understand the results of genetic testing and to make informed decisions about the next steps, which may include medical recommendations, additional testing, and the management of long-term cancer risk.

CHAPTER 6

The prevention of cancer and the treatment of cancer risk

The influence of genetics on the progression of cancer can be mitigated in part by taking preventative measures and actively managing one's cancer risk. When it comes to the prevention of cancer and the management of cancer risk, some important factors to consider include the following:

1. Changes in lifestyle Making changes to one's lifestyle, such as adopting a healthy diet, engaging in regular physical activity, and staying away from tobacco products and drinking an excessive amount of alcohol, can help lower one's risk of developing cancer.

2. Cancer screenings Having routine cancer screenings such as mammograms, colonoscopies, and pap smears can assist in

the early detection of cancer, which is the stage at which it is most amenable to treatment.

3. Surgery to reduce the risk of cancer: In certain circumstances, surgery may be recommended to remove organs or tissues that have a high risk of developing cancer. One example of this is a prophylactic mastectomy, which is performed on women who have a high risk of developing breast cancer.

4. Chemoprevention: Taking anti-cancer drugs like raloxifene or tamoxifen in order to lower one's chances of developing certain forms of cancer is referred to as chemoprevention.

5. Monitoring and surveillance Consistent monitoring and surveillance, which may include imaging tests and physical exams, can assist in the early detection of cancer and the monitoring for recurrence of the disease.

6. Access to support and resources: Having access to support and resources, such as genetic counseling, cancer support groups, and mental health services, can assist individuals and families in coping with the emotional and psychological impact of a cancer diagnosis and the risk of developing cancer.

It is essential to develop a personalized plan for the prevention and management of cancer risk in collaboration with a trained medical professional. This plan should include regular cancer screenings, risk-reducing strategies, and ongoing monitoring and surveillance.

Steps that can be taken to reduce the risk of cancer based on genetic information

1. Gain an understanding of your family's cancer history. Gaining an understanding of

your family's cancer history can provide valuable insights into your own risk of developing cancer. Gather information from close relatives about the type of cancer, the age at which symptoms first appeared, and any other pertinent details.

2. Get tested: If someone in your family has had cancer or if you have other risk factors, you should seriously consider getting genetic testing to assess your likelihood of developing cancer. This information can assist you in making educated decisions regarding the screening, prevention, and management of cancer.

3. Make changes to your lifestyle Some lifestyle factors, such as diet, physical activity, and avoiding tobacco and excessive alcohol consumption, can have an impact on the risk of developing cancer. Altering any of these behaviors can assist in lowering the risk you face.

4. Give thought to getting screened for cancer Depending on the severity of your cancer risk, you may need to get screened for cancer more frequently or at an earlier age. This can detect cancer in its earliest stages, when it is also the easiest to treat.

5. Reduce your risk of disease through medical treatment If the results of your genetic test indicate that you have an increased risk of cancer, you may be able to reduce that risk through medical treatment. This may involve the use of medication, surgical procedures, or some other kind of treatment.

6. Continue to educate yourself: Continue to educate yourself on the latest advances in cancer genetics and risk management. Review your family history and risk factors on a regular basis, and if you have any concerns, talk to your healthcare provider about them.

7. Be an advocate for yourself and your health by arming yourself with knowledge about the genetics of cancer and speaking up for yourself. This includes actively advocating for your own health and well-being as well as seeking out reputable information sources, keeping up with the latest developments in the field, and staying informed about those advancements.

You will be able to use your genetic information to make educated decisions about your potential cancer risk and take steps to reduce that risk if you follow these steps. It is essential to keep in mind that not all cancers are caused by genetics, and that other factors, such as lifestyle and environmental exposures, can also play a role in the development of the disease.

Using one's genetic information, strategies for reducing one's risk of developing cancer

In order to reduce the risk of cancer based on genetic information, one must take measures to either prevent or manage the impact that genetic mutations have on the development of cancer. The following are some important considerations to make:

1. Gaining an understanding of genetic mutations Gaining an understanding of the specific genetic mutations that increase the risk for cancer can help contribute to the formation of decisions regarding the management and prevention of cancer.

2. Alterations to one's lifestyle Making changes to one's lifestyle that are healthy, such as maintaining a healthy diet, getting regular exercise, and avoiding tobacco and excessive alcohol consumption, can assist in lowering one's risk of developing cancer.

3. Routine cancer screenings Having routine cancer screenings, such as mammograms, colonoscopies, and pap smears, can assist in

the early detection of cancer, when it is at its most treatable stage.

4. Surgery to reduce the risk of cancer: In some instances, surgery may be recommended to remove organs or tissues that have a high risk of developing cancer. For example, a preventative mastectomy may be recommended for women who have a high risk of developing breast cancer.

5. Chemoprevention: Taking anti-cancer drugs like raloxifene or tamoxifen in order to lower one's chances of developing certain forms of cancer is one method of chemoprevention.

6. Monitoring and surveillance Consistent monitoring and surveillance, which may include imaging tests and physical exams, can assist in the early detection of cancer and the monitoring for recurrence of the disease.

7. Access to support and resources: Having access to support and resources, such as genetic counseling, cancer support groups, and mental health services, can assist individuals and families in coping with the emotional and psychological impact of a cancer diagnosis and the risk of developing cancer.

It is important to work with a medical professional to develop a personalized plan for reducing cancer risk based on genetic information. This plan should include ongoing monitoring and surveillance, regular cancer screenings, and risk-reducing strategies.

How to reduce the risk of cancer through adjustments in one's lifestyle as well as through medical treatment

Modifying one's lifestyle and receiving medical treatment can be helpful in lowering one's risk of developing cancer. As part of this process, one must take measures to prevent or lessen the effect that genetic mutations have on the development of cancer. The following are some important considerations to keep in mind:

1. Changes in lifestyle Making changes to one's lifestyle, such as adopting a healthy diet, engaging in regular physical activity, and staying away from tobacco products and drinking an excessive amount of alcohol, can help lower one's risk of developing cancer.

2. Cancer screenings Having routine cancer screenings such as mammograms, colonoscopies, and pap smears can assist in the early detection of cancer, which is the stage at which it is most amenable to treatment.

3. Surgery to reduce the risk of cancer: In certain circumstances, surgery may be

recommended to remove organs or tissues that have a high risk of developing cancer. One example of this is a prophylactic mastectomy, which is performed on women who have a high risk of developing breast cancer.

4. Chemoprevention: Taking anti-cancer drugs like raloxifene or tamoxifen in order to lower one's chances of developing certain forms of cancer is referred to as chemoprevention.

5. Monitoring and surveillance Consistent monitoring and surveillance, which may include imaging tests and physical exams, can assist in the early detection of cancer and the monitoring for recurrence of the disease.

6. Access to support and resources: Having access to support and resources, such as genetic counseling, cancer support groups,

and mental health services, can assist individuals and families in coping with the emotional and psychological impact of a cancer diagnosis and the risk of developing cancer.

It is essential to develop a personalized plan for managing cancer risk through lifestyle changes and medical intervention with the help of a medical professional.
This plan should include regular cancer screenings, risk-reducing strategies, and ongoing monitoring and surveillance. Individuals may be better able to take charge of their cancer risk and make decisions that are more beneficial to their health with the help of this approach.

A complete list of the various screening and preventative measures available for cancer

There are numerous cancer screening and prevention options available; these options vary depending on the type of cancer and the specific risk factors of the individual. The following is an outline of some of the more common methods of cancer screening and prevention:

1. Cancer screenings Having routine cancer screenings, such as mammograms, colonoscopies, and pap smears, can assist in the early detection of cancer, which is the stage at which it is the most amenable to treatment.

2. Genetic testing Individuals who are at an increased risk for certain types of cancer can be identified through genetic testing. This paves the way for earlier and more frequent cancer screenings as well as other preventative measures.

3. Alterations to one's lifestyle Making changes to one's lifestyle that are healthy, such as maintaining a healthy diet, getting

regular exercise, and avoiding tobacco and excessive alcohol consumption, can assist in lowering one's risk of developing cancer.

4. Chemoprevention: Taking anti-cancer drugs like raloxifene or tamoxifen in order to lower one's chances of developing certain forms of cancer is referred to as chemoprevention.

5. Surgery to reduce the risk of cancer: In some instances, surgery may be recommended to remove organs or tissues that have a high risk of developing cancer.
For example, a preventative mastectomy may be recommended for women who have a high risk of developing breast cancer.

6. Vaccines: Some vaccines, like the one for human papillomavirus (HPV), have been shown to reduce the risk of developing certain cancers.

7. Monitoring and surveillance Routine monitoring and surveillance, which may include imaging tests and physical exams, can assist in the early detection of cancer and the monitoring for recurrence of the disease.

In order to determine the cancer screening and prevention options that are best suited for an individual, taking into account their unique set of risk factors and medical history, it is essential to collaborate with a trained medical professional. Cancer screenings and other preventative actions, when performed on a regular basis, can help lower the risk of developing cancer and increase the likelihood of detecting it at an early stage, when it is at its most treatable.

CHAPTER 7

Conclusion

The writers of The Power of Genes: Understanding Cancer Risk Through Genetics provide an inference in which they summarize the most important points discussed throughout the book and stress the significance of having an understanding of the role that genetics play in determining cancer risk. They highlight the benefits of genetic testing and family history analysis in helping individuals understand their own cancer risk and take steps to reduce that risk through changes in lifestyle, medical interventions, and cancer screening and prevention options. These benefits are highlighted in the article.

The authors also emphasize how important it is to consult with a qualified medical professional in order to comprehend the repercussions of the findings of genetic testing and to make educated decisions regarding the management of cancer risk. They encourage people to educate themselves about the influence that genetics have on their risk of developing cancer and to be proactive in taking steps to reduce that risk of developing cancer in their own bodies.

In the final chapter of the book, the author issues a rallying cry to readers, urging them to take charge of their own health and collaborate with the professionals who care for them in order to better understand and control their potential for developing cancer.

A synopsis of the most important lessons learned from the book

The following is a list of the most important things that I learned from reading The Power of Genes: Understanding Cancer Risk Through Genetics:
1. A person's family history is an important factor in determining their cancer risk, and

having a good understanding of one's family tree is essential to making an accurate assessment of that risk.

2. Breast and ovarian cancer are two of the many types of cancer that have been associated with the BRCA1 and BRCA2 genes, which are two genes that have been linked to an increased risk of developing cancer.

3. The history of one's family is an important aspect to consider when estimating one's likelihood of developing cancer; the gathering and examination of information regarding one's family history can assist in the identification of individuals who are at an elevated risk for certain cancers.

4. Although genetic testing can provide useful information about a person's risk of developing cancer, prior to undergoing testing, one should carefully consider the potential psychological and physical repercussions that the test results may have.

5. Adopting a healthier way of life by avoiding risky behaviors like smoking and drinking to excess, as well as keeping a healthy diet and not overindulging in alcohol, can help lower one's risk of developing cancer.

6. Regular cancer screenings, medical interventions, and preventive measures can help reduce the risk of developing cancer and detect cancer at an earlier stage.

7. Individuals and their healthcare providers should collaborate to understand the implications of the results of their genetic tests and make decisions about the management of their cancer risk that are based on accurate information.

This book provides a comprehensive overview of the role that genetics play in cancer risk as well as the steps that individuals can take to reduce their own risk of developing cancer. The book is titled "The Power of Genes: Understanding Cancer Risk Through Genetics." Individuals are able to take charge of their health and make educated decisions regarding the management of their cancer risk when they have a thorough understanding of their genetic background and collaborate with their healthcare providers.

Final thoughts; on the role that genes play in determining the risk of developing cancer

There is no denying the significance that genetics plays in the process of understanding cancer risk. Individuals can gain valuable insights into their risk and take steps to reduce that risk if they are aware of their genetic background and the role that it plays in determining their risk of developing certain types of cancer. Genetics plays a significant role in determining an individual's risk of developing certain types of cancer.

An individual's potential cancer risk can be significantly reduced by obtaining information about their family medical history, conducting an analysis of that information, and undergoing genetic testing. Individuals are able to reduce their risk of developing cancer by making changes to their lifestyle, undergoing medical interventions, and taking advantage of various cancer screening and prevention options if they collaborate with the healthcare providers who are responsible for their care.

It is essential to keep in mind that the hereditary predisposition to cancer is only one factor in determining the likelihood of developing the disease; environmental and lifestyle factors also play a significant role. However, if a person is aware of the role that their genes play in their likelihood of developing cancer, they are better equipped to make educated choices regarding their health and to collaborate with the professionals who care for them to lower their likelihood of developing the disease.

In conclusion, the power of genetics in the understanding of cancer risk is a valuable tool for individuals who are looking to take control of their health and reduce the risk that they will develop cancer. Individuals are able to make educated decisions about the management of their cancer risk and the steps they should take to reduce that risk when they collaborate with their healthcare providers.

Definition of some terminologies used in this book

Here are definitions of some terminologies used in "The Power of Genes: Understanding Cancer Risk Through Genetics":

1. Cancer genetics: the study of the role of genetics in the development and progression of cancer.

2. Cancer risk: the likelihood of developing cancer, which can be influenced by a variety of factors including genetics, lifestyle, and environmental factors.
3. Genetic mutations: changes or alterations in the DNA sequence that can lead to changes in the function of a gene.
4. Inherited mutations: mutations that are passed down from a parent to a child.
5. Acquired mutations: mutations that occur during a person's lifetime and are not passed down from a parent.
6. Family history: a record of medical conditions and diseases that have occurred in a person's family, including cancers.
7. Genetic testing: the analysis of a person's DNA to determine the presence or absence of specific genetic mutations.
8. Cancer screening: the use of tests or procedures to detect cancer in its early stages, when it is most treatable.
9. Prevention: measures taken to reduce the risk of developing cancer, such as lifestyle changes and medical intervention.
10. Management: the process of monitoring and treating cancer risk, including cancer screening and prevention measures.

11. BRCA1 gene: a gene that provides instructions for making a protein that helps suppress the growth of tumor cells. Mutations in this gene are associated with an increased risk of certain cancers, including breast and ovarian cancer.
12. BRCA2 gene: a gene that provides instructions for making a protein that helps suppress the growth of tumor cells. Mutations in this gene are associated with an increased risk of certain cancers, including breast and prostate cancer.
13. Lifestyle changes: changes to one's habits and behaviors, such as exercise and diet, that can help reduce cancer risk.
14. Medical intervention: medical treatments or procedures used to reduce cancer risk, such as surgery, radiation therapy, and chemotherapy.
15. Cancer syndromes: conditions in which a person is at an increased risk of developing certain types of cancer due to an inherited genetic mutation.
16. Genetic information: information about a person's genetic makeup, including genetic mutations and family history.
17. Healthcare providers: medical professionals, such as doctors and nurses,

who provide healthcare services to patients.

18. Environmental factors: elements in the environment that can impact cancer risk, such as exposure to harmful chemicals or pollutants.

19. Cancer research: scientific study aimed at understanding the causes of cancer and developing new treatments.

20. Patient advocacy: the act of advocating on behalf of patients, including advocating for access to information and resources related to cancer genetics.

21. Genetic resources: resources, such as books, websites, and support groups, that provide information and support related to genetics and cancer.

www.ingramcontent.com/pod-product-compliance
Lightning Source LLC
Chambersburg PA
CBHW071142220526
45467CB00015B/1709